# My Transformation…

## The real truth about Weight Loss Surgery

My story

## Disclaimer

scanning, mechanical or recording without prior written permission from the author.

While the author has taken utmost efforts to ensure the accuracy of the written content, all readers are advised to follow the information mentioned herein at their own risk. The author cannot be held responsible for any personal or commercial damage caused by misinterpretation of information. All readers are encouraged to seek professional advice when needed.

This e-book has been written for information purposes only. Every effort has been made to make this eBook as complete and accurate as possible. However, there may be mistakes in typography or content. Also, this e-book provides information only up to the publishing date. Therefore, this eBook should be used as a guide - not as the ultimate source.

The author and the publisher do not warrant that the information contained in this e-book is fully complete and shall not be responsible for any errors or omissions. The author and publisher shall have neither liability nor responsibility to any person or entity with respect to any loss or damage caused or alleged to be caused directly or indirectly by this e-book.

# Table of Contents

# Introduction

With the number of obese people increasing each year, there are now billions of people who can be classified as being overweight. As per the findings of the World Health Organisation (WHO), in 2014, the number of overweight adults touched 1.9 billion. Among whom, 600 million could be classified as obese. The most optimistic thought about this figure can only be the assumption that it has only *doubled* by now and not more than that!

According to the World Health Organisation, individuals with a Body Mass Index of greater than or equal to 25 are considered overweight while individuals with a Body Mass Index of greater than or equal to 30 are considered obese!

Being overweight can have various reasons, such as overeating, lack of exercise and a proper lifestyle, genetic predisposition, lack of sleep, poor nutrition, eating disorders, and medication side effects. People tend to not care much when they eat more than they should, but they begin to do so when they are met with the consequences!

Overweight people, in fact, have an inversely proportional relationship with life expectancy. Being overweight is also linked to dangerous diseases like cancers, and diabetes. While this information will nudge you in the right direction, let us not forget that obesity may also result in severe heart diseases. Besides the problems that you face internally, many of us are also subjected to social stigma and fat shaming on a daily basis.

Loving yourself the way you are is very important. But have you ever seen a spoiled child, for whom every wish and whim has been fulfilled? For whom generosity and kindness begin to cause more harm than good? This is what I believe is generally happening when people foster the idea of loving their fat bodies. By no means do I want to judge or fat shame anyone. But truth be told, a line needs to be drawn. We all should realize if we are close to touching that line before it is too late. Achieving happiness in our own bodies and minds is crucial!

# Chapter 1: The Beginning of My Weight Loss Journey

It is empowering for me to say it out loud that yes, I have shed a lot of weight. The feeling that I get when I put it into writing is completely indescribable. It is indeed an accolade to achieve your desired weight. I was hugely obese. Yeah, it is all in the past now; it has become a memory since I took a massive and significant step. I did that before it was too late and everything would get out of hand.

I lived a normal life like any other UK resident. A thirty-two-year-old woman, a wife, a career-oriented female, and a mother of two beautiful girls – both under the age of three – in short, I was an average, everyday woman.

With a height of 5 ft. and 7 inches, my body weighed around 159 kg or approx. 25 stones. I had inhabited this obese body for so long it never occurred to me that it was a problem. Or maybe, I was too blind to realize it. The only thing that I remembered was that I had been carrying this pile of fat for many, many years.

My life was centred on other important people – my husband, my girls, family, and my job. By no means did I find time to think about my weight, or that's what I told myself. My mind always fostered the idea that I *should* love myself the way I was, but deep down, I knew that I could look better.

Whenever I would see a slim woman, I would ask myself what it would be like, to be slim... But this was only limited to my thoughts, and I would never dedicate much time to it, nor would I take it personally. As long as I was able to please the people I loved, it didn't matter to me, too much, how I looked or what I weighed.

I was constantly telling myself that I couldn't achieve it, and, that I shouldn't take it personally; it was 'ok'. Giving it deep thought would have shown me that I really did want to achieve that slimmer me. I wanted to wake up one day and see myself in the mirror as a regular Jo, just minus the fat that surrounded me. I wanted to be the fit mommy whose daughters would be proud of her. The mom whom they could take to any school function without getting ashamed. This is what I thought, even though my daughters and my husband didn't care about my appearance and weight.

Once I had those thoughts, I would begin telling myself that these things weren't even related. I should not care about these things, but I did. Deep down I did care, and the thought of it had started becoming unbearable over time. As my babies were growing up, I began to think about this more often.

The process of becoming obese is not like a potion that you can drink and gain weight overnight. Neither it is like only waking up and realizing that you are fat like due to a magic spell or an extra treat. The process takes time. It sneaks into your life every day of the week and every week of the month and so on! You only realize when it's beyond the phase of **"It cannot be ignored anymore!"** It is also what happened to me!

From what I remember, I wasn't that overweight in the early days of my youth, but as I entered my late teenage years, I just grew taller and wider.

Like a parasite that lives off the host without the host realizing its existence, obesity slid into my life. Or, in polite terms, like a harmless insect in a flower pot, bound to harm you, and do much more but is noticeable only if you pay attention to the insect. Otherwise, it just keeps growing inside.

During our childhood days, we all are told that it's all 'puppy fat' and we will get rid of it as we grow up. Most people actually lose weight, but I don't think they do so naturally. Maybe it is due to the fact that they realized it before it was too late?

When I was an overweight teenager, I did absolutely nothing to stop it, and maybe everything to aggravate it. I always had lots of friends at school although I was classified as a 'big' girl. I always felt good about myself and was popular. Thus, I did nothing to change it. I was always hopeful that I would change in the future somehow whenever I wanted to.

I also learned a good proverb that is, "You sow so should you reap!" So, that extra slice of cake, that triple sandwich, the donut AND waffles with cream, and the cheesy fries – they all kept on showing their traces years after being gobbled. And I did nothing. They presented themselves in the form of fat and in the form of flab. Even so, I was always under the impression that I was just 'big' and not really fat. Since I was also tall, I carried it well.

I have learned to accept a trait associated with my personality – I am indeed just *greedy!* Everyone has some kind of vice and food was always mine. However, with very little help or persuasion, I will embark on a journey to get what I strive for. I would always go that extra mile in most of what mattered in my life and in all that I did and still do. I like to live life on the edge, and it is hard and nearly impossible for me to disregard or abandon what I strive for. I think I'm driven with, what most would call, stubbornness!!

Food was something I craved for more than money or possessions.

Once I started eating, I'd take number of huge spoonful, one after another, just to find out that the plate was empty. If I wanted a Mars bar, I would buy one for eating now and keep one to eat later. There was nothing stopping me with food, so why should I not eat what I wanted to? Food was, and still is something divine and wholesome for me. Back then, I used to think that if I could have 1, why not have 3? Pure greed, I know! My wonderful sister reminded me of this a while back when I was talking and moaning about being so unfortunate in my younger days to be fat, and why it had happened to me. She reminded me that I was simply just GREEDY, not 'unfortunate' and we chuckled – she was right, of course.

My love for food was silently killing me and I was letting it do so, and enjoying it way, way too much...

Sometimes, I would see my reflection in the windows of the shops down the street and would tell myself, Joanne, something needs to be done about this. You will have to get rid of the flab! I think the fat also made me look older and quite frumpy, but as a teenager, I didn't mind looking older either. Looking older was 'cool', however, my thoughts would then increase my enthusiasm to lose weight and I would start working on it. For some time, I would try anything, just to see some kind of results.

I joined gyms, went running and swimming for a short period of time until I got bored, or hungry.

I followed various diet gurus, zero-eating days, various slimming clubs, liquid diets, and shakes. I even tried the Cabbage diet and the Atkins diet. Despite my love for food, I would take different combinations of fruits and vegetables just to adjust the calorie count – let's highlight one more thing here; they all tasted utterly disgusting and not sustainable.

Occasionally, I would even lose a few pounds and sometimes up to 6 kg (1 stone) at a time. But the problem was, that if I missed just a single day of diet food, my entire motivation would break and I would be back to consuming the same unhealthy and gorgeously rich food. Not only would I gain the lost pounds, but I would pile on a few more. It was like a cycle; I would lose a few lbs., then become bored with it, miss on just a single day, and be back to the same old detrimental eating habits. As a result, I would gain extra layers of fat after every failed attempt. But being tall, I hid it well.

This cycle continued for years since I was not completely ready to let go of my favourite foods and adopt healthy eating habits. I found it really hard to survive on tasteless food… With time, though, I learned one thing that I shall forever stay overweight and that no one can help me if I didn't help myself.

Easier said than done though because I would do the housework, sort out the kids' stuff, go to work, and after everything, I would have little time left for myself. When I joined a gym, the sweat and pain just irritated me. Even if I would make some kind of progress in the gym, I would later meet my friends, consume drinks, and gorge on takeaways – and guess what happened next? I was soon off from the diet!

The exercise wasn't for me and I hated it to the core! Apparently, I had forgotten all about losing weight, but reality hit me hard in the face. It came in front of me in a way that I couldn't ignore it in any way, anymore!

I was changing my elder daughter's nappy (aged 2) while my younger daughter (aged 1) began to cry in the bedroom upstairs. In a rush, to attend to her, I tried to get up, but alas! I just couldn't. No matter how much I tried, I failed, and I failed badly. I was like a wet fish, flapping about on the floor, struggling to get up!

I had never realized that I had brought myself to this state of mortal peril and shame. I was becoming immovable; I couldn't get up by myself and I ached everywhere.

I looked into my daughter's eyes and burst into tears. I was also thinking about the many types of fatal medical conditions I could get – any of them would leave my kids without a mother!

That was it! That very moment was the time when I swore to put an end to it. I promised myself that there will be no running away from reality. I promised myself that I will up my health game for the sake of the people I love, not just for cosmetic reasons, but for the sake of retaining my health in the long run!

The Internet was my first refuge. I began to search about losing weight online. I was beyond embarrassed to discuss this with any of my friends, which is why I had opted for virtual help.

The internet helped me embark on the first step of this journey. That step was to accept my decision! Acceptance – yeah, I had already accepted the way my body was, but I couldn't muster the courage for the next step.

The second step was to convince myself to work on weight reduction and achieve body fitness. I didn't seek temporary results but sought for the ones that would last in the future.

I soon realized that I wasn't alone when it came to constant failure at losing weight. Honestly, it lessened my anxiety and made me feel relieved. The information and the content I found were indeed overwhelming. However, following any of them thoroughly throughout each stage was cumbersome. I could see hundreds of different options that were available for me to try – each of them came with different risks and costs.

As mentioned before, working out at the gym was certainly not my thing. I would be sometimes motivated by watching those weight loss videos, but that sudden rush in the adrenaline wouldn't keep me going for long.

Clean eating wouldn't do it alone; I knew that! Jogging and exercising were not something that my body would be able to take for too long. So the only option (I thought) I was left with, was, surgery. I believed that only if someone else cuts the fat off me, then I would be able to see a slimmer me. It wasn't something that I could achieve by myself though. I wanted it done quickly; quick results would keep me motivated. I can see now how that was quite a naïve way of thinking.

I reviewed literally everything, from jaw wiring to stomach stapling. I read the most dreadful articles and I watched the most cringe-worthy videos – the ultimate goal was to find a solution for me to get rid of the flab and extra pounds.

I investigated and researched rigorously. It finally boiled down to the following three options for my fat reduction surgery. These options were: the Roux-en-Y (RNY), the Gastric Band, and the Duodenal Switch (DS); all quite costly options.

**Get ready for the medical information**

RNY, also known as a form of the 'Gastric Bypass' is the procedure in which your stomach is divided into two parts. One is much smaller than the other part. This is called a pouch and can hold only a small amount of food, and thus, would make you feel full after eating only a tiny portion of food.

Besides this, the Gastric bypass also helps in reducing the absorption of calories and nutrients. The smaller stomach is disconnected from the larger one and also from the duodenum. It is then directly attached to the jejunum; this surgical technique is called Roux-en-Y. It helps in sufficient weight reduction with minimal "malabsorption."

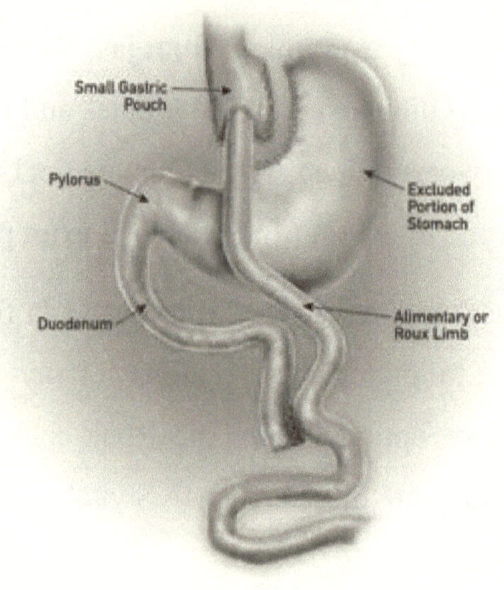




The second option, the gastric band involves the placement of a silicone band around the upper part of the stomach to divide the stomach into two chambers. The upper chamber has a narrow opening that restricts food to pass down to the second chamber.

The band can be adjusted to control the amount of food that passes – it can either be relaxed or tightened to meet the food passing restrictions. Thus, the band helps in controlling your cravings and eventually impacts your weight loss regime.

The band is inflated or deflated to reduce or increase the space in the upper chamber of your stomach and forms an effective control on the food intake.

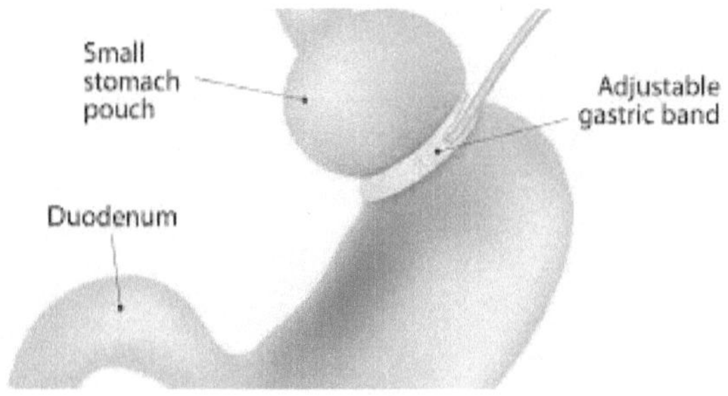



Source: https://www.yourbariatricsurgeryguide.com/gastric-banding/

The third option was the duodenal switch. DS was the most physically intrusive option. It is sometimes referred to as Sleeve gastrostomy. It has both, the mal-absorptive and the restrictive aspects. A full DS procedure removes approximately 70% of the patient's stomach. Also, it will bypass two third of the small intestines.

One of its parts, the alimentary limb is connected to the stomach while the other part, the biliopancreatic limb performs the function of keeping the digestive juices away from the gall bladder and the pancreas until the common point of meeting approaches. This prevents the body from absorbing excess calories and fat, and, thus aids **significantly** in losing weight. The DS guaranteed the most weight loss out of all three procedures, but it was also obviously the most intrusive and dangerous.

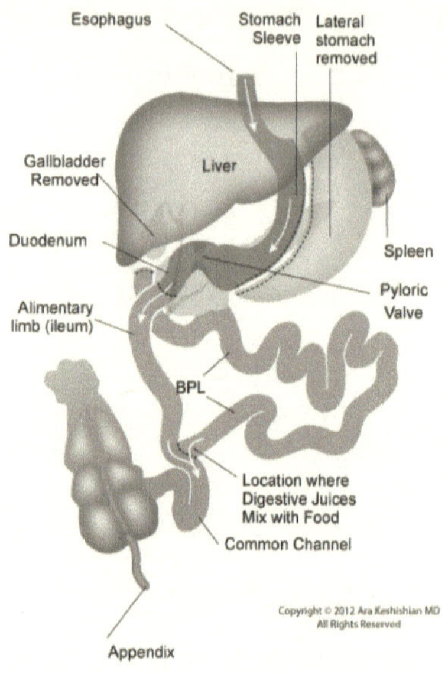



Source: https://www.dssurgery.com/weight-loss-surgery/laparoscopic-duodenal-switch/

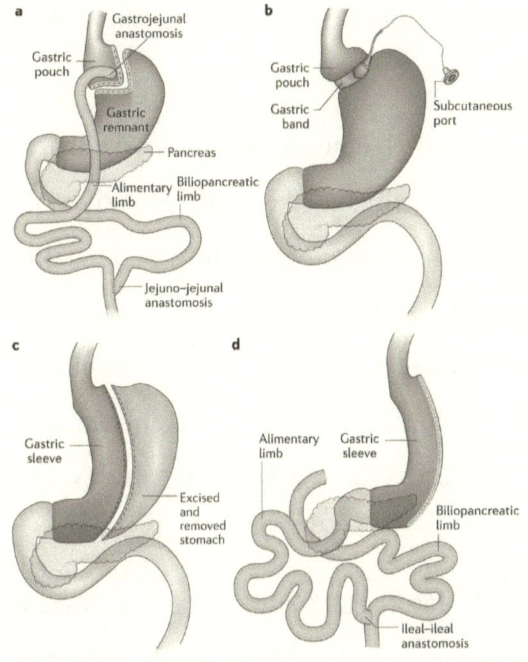


Source: https://www.nature.com/articles/nrgastro.2016.170/figures/1

With this information in hand, I had to make some decisions.

The first option to be crossed off the list was the gastric band. I felt that I would have to work too hard with this one, and it guaranteed the least amount of weight loss. Also, I wanted fast results while the gastric band would have taken more time.

The next best option was the RNY; it offered 60% of guaranteed weight loss. But again, I wanted a 100% fat-free body! Hence, the only option left was the duodenal switch DS.

Without any initial consultation, I knew that it was my body's only saviour and the most effective of the three. However, it came with complexities, high health risks, and the highest rate of fatalities. It was something that I had chosen for myself and I would think about the downside only later. Obviously, I wanted to see instantaneous results where possible; maybe I was setting my expectations too high.

Note that with fewer calorie absorption, it was also implied that fewer nutrients and vitamins would be absorbed by my body. But that wasn't a concern of mine at this early stage. Shedding extra weight was the prime focus for me. What I wanted were prompt and positive results, but only in terms of weight reduction!

I wanted to get rid of that ugly, troublesome, and undesirable body – ANY WAY I COULD and FAST!!!

Without giving a second thought to the clinical or psychological effects it carried, I actually became excited about the results. I knew that it would involve a lot of sacrifices. That it would involve a lot of adaptation and physical, mental, and psychological healing, but I had just one answer to all of it – BRING IT ON! I was so excited.

Why was I so oblivious, you might ask? Think about what life was like for me each day. I would check out myself in the mirror, all naked, and ashamed of myself. It got me angry, irritated, and disgusted. I looked much older than my years, frumpy, and fat. I had almost killed myself out of stubbornness and had turned my beautiful body into an undesirable and uglier one – just out of my lust for food and lack of exercise. Not anymore, I told myself, not anymore!

I wanted to see immediate results, with zero disappointment, and I wanted no one to tell me to hold off or to slow down! Even if someone had told me to get rid of a few bones that I didn't need just to achieve the weight reduction, I would have gladly done so!

No one else was in my shoes, so they couldn't really understand.

With the passage of time, I was becoming more excited about having a flab-free body. In elaborated terms, I had become obsessed with the thought of shedding the weight. This was like awakening from ignorance. A light had turned on in my head, and nothing could put me to sleep anymore.

My thoughts would often wander to how my daughters will regard me when they grow up? I had started envying the slim and trim women around me. Then, a second thought that struck me was that just like I envied them, what would they think about me? Would they frown upon my weight, or whisper under their breath?

I began to have serious concerns about it myself. A friend said 'how someone maintains himself tells much about them as a person'. We all should prioritise ourselves, and if we are not bothered about our own appearance, then we really do not have that "substance and self-worth." This resonated with me.

I was longing to see the surgeon who could help. I finally landed myself with an appointment scheduled with an amazing bariatric surgeon in the UK. We'll call him Sam. I was anticipating to have a long drawn conversation with him about how we can go about the procedure, and how it will affect my body positively.

I was looking forward for him to register me for a duodenal switch procedure as soon as possible. But to my amazement, his answer to my statement, "I have to get rid of all of this fat!" was, "My advice for you is to do the RNY procedure, not DS."

Sam told me to go for an RNY! Just because I kept myself calm and didn't allow my excitement of losing weight to be seen through my words, he had told me to go for an option. It would yield slightly lesser results but would be better for my body in the long run.

"But I prefer the DS," I had to interrupt him with this! He didn't pay much attention, just nodded. He then asked me a few more questions to assess my health. This made me even more anxious. I had already made up my mind on to its direction; nothing was swaying me.

Prompt, fast, and effective, that is what could define the duodenal switch for me. I wanted something that would wash off all the traces of fat and the traces of cellulite.

Sam, my surgeon, tried to advise me otherwise. His major decision was the fact that **I was much lighter** than a patient who is recommended a duodenal switch. Because of that, the risks associated with an RNY were much lower than with a duodenal switch. He didn't want me to take on this additional challenge on my body. He shook his head as he explained all of this to me.

My heart began to sink. I felt like I was moving away from my weight loss goals. I knew that the RNY has lesser risks associated with it, but it also brought about a lesser EWL (estimated weight loss)!

"It would not give me my desired weight reduction!" my voice reflected the disappointment I was feeling. "If my only way of getting the DS was by being heavier, then okay, I will be back in a couple of months. I'd be heavier then, I explained. I will eat all I can, and do all I can to get heavier and meet the weight requirements for the DS. And then I would get the surgery I want!"

I assured him I was very determined and that I will go that extra mile to get him to agree to let me opt for the duodenal switch procedure.

He must have thought that I was crazy. I know I would have thought that too if I had been in his place. But I wasn't, so did I care? No, I did not. I knew what I wanted and I was stubborn as ever. I only saw my goal going further miles away if I didn't insist on DS. Nothing else matters, I explained to the doctor!

I knew deep down that I was someone who was determined, and even if something is detrimental to me, I don't give a thought about its aftermath and consequences.

The only thing I would care about is my ultimate goal. Obviously, I didn't share that information with him...

My fat body was looking worse by the day. I wanted to get rid of the fat in any way I could. If magic spells could do it, I would have tried them. Anything was okay with me since I had an ideal picture in my mind. When you want something so badly, that is how you behave. Anything that takes you further away from the goal wouldn't do. I wanted to bridge the gap between reality and my imagination at any price.

The person to whom I owe much during my entire weight loss journey was my then husband. He understood me more than anyone else, he could relate to my circumstances, being larger himself at the time. He understood what I was enduring, physically, emotionally, and socially.

I didn't want to be the centre of all mockery by the mothers' of my children's friends once they began their schooling. Being called "the old fat mom in the schoolyard!" was my biggest nightmare. Children tend to follow their parents' footsteps. Now was a good time to have the surgery while mine were still young as it wouldn't have major implications on their values. It would have broken my heart if my daughter would ever come back home crying after she had been bullied because of me.

Moving into my thirties, I had to set things right. Okay, I admit that I was being a lunatic and entirely dogmatic, but, I needed it so much. My husband and I talked about it in depth.

"Are you sure you want to do this?" he had asked me. "Yes, I want to do this." To the maximum was my reply.

"This surgery means the world to me. I wanted to be normal in size and this will change me, make me better." I added, he didn't look convinced but agreed.

He nodded. I think he needed confidence in me that I knew what I had chosen and I had researched it well.

We re-mortgaged our house to raise the money for the surgery. We had to get the money somehow.

I did not want to regret anything in the future, so I took the step that was necessary, rather than taking a loan or using credit cards.

I was already excited at how I was paving my way towards my goal. However, I didn't realize, the re-mortgage was only the first challenge that we would tackle. Many more of them were on the way. I am not only talking in monetary terms but emotional, physical, and psychological challenges as well.

However, I was determined. I was determined to make the most of this opportunity, for the best of all of us.

I'm aware of the fact that you have to sacrifice something in order to get something in return, but if I thought that sailing my boat in this storm would be painless and trouble free, how wrong I was!

~End of chapter 1~

# Chapter 2: OMG! It is finally happening!

After re-mortgaging the house and using part of our savings, we had paid a huge amount to make my weight reduction dream a reality. Not yet a fact, but my dream was in the making. My hero, my surgeon Sam, had asked me to wait 6 weeks. He also advised me to lose 5 kg before my body went under the knife, this was standard.

The time span made me even more anxious. I wanted it all to happen so swiftly, but now I had to wait again. This time it was not for days, but for SIX WEEKS!

I felt I was so close, and yet so far away. Everything was set in place, but the only factor that posed a hurdle in my way was the time – and losing 5kg. Each day seemed to be longer than the one before. Like the grain of sands going down the hourglass gradually, my days passed slowly. Each day made me excited as I would mark it off the calendar.

I would dream about it every day and do anything to make the time pass – literally! However, losing 5 kg was very difficult for me. Each meal that I had, seemed like the last. I finally got there and lost the full 5 Kg. I was ready.

The big day approached us after much anticipation. I remember having my last big meal before the surgical procedure and waking up full of enthusiasm the next morning. Everything was on target. The money had been deposited, the 5 kg had been shed, and I was now ready.

The excitement began to take the face of fear and hesitance as the hospital got nearer. With just a short 1-hour car ride, my heart began to thump in my chest. I had studied so much about the procedure and results, and yet I was still nervous. I wondered if it would work the same for me and if I'd have any complications. It had been so long with all these layers of fat that it was hard to think about not having this fat on my bones in the near future.

The fear of something awful happening began to creep into my mind. My subconscious mind came up with one of the worst scenarios that could occur during the operation.

What if I bled beyond the normal level and the hospital was not able to arrange blood for me? What if my heart stopped beating and I lay lifeless on the operation table? What if... what if…

I had horrendous thoughts running through my mind. Yet, I was also excited about it. The factors that should have been considered by me before had begun to haunt me now. My thoughts began to wander around what would happen if the surgery did not work out for me, despite paying huge sums of money and putting my family and friends through such an ordeal.

Not only did I take the risk, but the people I love were also made to endure the stress and had to go through the emotional labour to see me in pain and discomfort. It was not easy for my husband to let me undergo this surgery. Be that as it may, the duodenal switch has also proven fatal for a few, and yes, my body was to be subjected to all those risks.

I couldn't exactly imagine that the ton of fat that I see will be no more, however, I hoped that that would be true soon.

I wasn't sure if the money that we had paid would be justified and how long would it take before we noticed any kind of difference. Will my family and I be able to cope with my unpredictable, unknown medical concerns? At this point, another question came into my mind: will it be even worth it? What if after everything, I was left unsatisfied?

I was waiting desperately for this day, and now that I was living it, it was full of doubts and negative thoughts. I told myself that it was just last minute nerves!

At that point, shame crept in! How on earth did I get here? The stage where I was risking my life in order to make it fat-free, when I had risked so much already, just to secure a thinner me. How did I even let things get this far? Why was I so ignorant and pig-headed?

I looked at myself in the mirror. Did I really hate the way my body was? YES!

Was I ready to go extra miles in order to secure weight reduction for myself? Yes! Definitely!

I reminded myself that I was not only doing it for myself but for the people whom I loved and the people who loved me. I wanted to stay around my girls and wanted to see them blossom and grow up. I wanted to see them happy in their lives, and I wanted to play with my grandchildren. Was that too much to ask for? No, I didn't think so.

Nothing should stop me from conquering this dream. The temporary pain was nothing in comparison to what the future held for me! There wasn't anything stopping me at that point.

I gave myself a pep-talk. I told myself that all would be fine. I told myself that it shall be worth it. Human beings don't fear the known, but we tend to only fear the unknown. The fear of the unknown had made me so worried and anxious.

I had immense support; so many people were waiting for me to come out healthy from the operation. I had to take this risk for a better tomorrow. I knew very little about what would happen afterward, but the risk of today was much better than the regrets of tomorrow.

I had read up various recovery stories of patients who had to undergo the same procedures as I was about to undergo and they were living a happy life.

I thought that I didn't want my girls to see me on the stretcher and ask several questions regarding it, so I had kissed them goodbye at home. I crossed my fingers and prayed to God not to make it our final goodbye.

I remember giving them a long, warm hug and suppressing my tears; I didn't want to get them worried. I didn't want them to think that I was going away, even for a second. My heart pounded as I told them that I was traveling for a few days. I didn't want this journey to become any more dramatic than it needed to be. Even for the few days, I was going to miss their laughter, their cries, their questions, and their mess! I was doing this so that my baby girls could be proud of me. So that they won't be ashamed at school gates and would not get bullied due to having a big fat mommy.

I had set forth on my journey toward the hospital. My husband tried to make a few jokes in order to relieve the tension, and I actually laughed. However, it didn't help in changing the way I felt. I knew that he was also tense; he was trying to cover up his emotions too.

I knew that I could still tell him to take me back and turnaround if needed, and I would not have to endure any of it, nor will my family. But no, this was it, and I would go through with it. The results would be too exciting!

No matter how scared I was, I had a clear vision of what I wanted and precisely what I needed. I was on the brink of creating a different life, to really make a difference for me that mattered.

I remember when I sat in a huge oversized chair, the nurse asked me to repeat my name several times as I was taken forward past the initial stages and I did so. Though I had been subjected to various blood tests in the past weeks, they took me to the laboratory for more. Blood screening had become a routine for me. My arms were so big that finding a vein became difficult for them. They screened my blood then proceeded with the medical checks.

They told my husband to leave. After that, I would be on my own. I would have to carry everything myself. I hugged him and didn't want to let him go, but I had to. I promised him that I would see him later with a big smile on my face. I was taken to the ward that was empty, apart from two patients who were fast asleep. Now the reality began to hit me on so many levels. I had to spend lonesome and painful days and nights in this place.

I was stripped naked and was told to wear the hospital big blue gown. I was then led to my own bed. The bed was hard, stiff, and crinkly; I knew the surgery in its entirety was not to provide a luxurious and comfortable experience. I waited for what was about to come. I waited, in excitement, and in terror.

I gazed at the ceilings and imagined myself thin, and tried to amuse myself in several ways. But nothing seemed to work. I was trying to keep myself immersed in positive thoughts, but I was failing. I had waited for hours already. The time that I had to kill before the anticipated procedure was the toughest. I had already begun to tremble.

But then the waiting time passed and I was like here we go...

I had already set foot into a new phase of my life. The things were all set to motion, and yes, it had started. After waiting for so many days, the time had finally come.

In the midst of boredom, a few nurses came to attend to me. They told me that it was time to begin with the procedures and we needed to go to the theatre soon. I actually couldn't waste any more time; I had to get it done and get over with it as soon as possible. I was taken to the operation theatre in a wheelchair with the doctors and nurses by my side.

Then in walked my surgeon, Sam! My ultimate hero. He had a lovely warm glow about him, like an angel. Sam was smart, but in no means scary, just warm, and soothing. He was nothing like I had expected him to be on surgery day. In fact, Sam was far more casual than he had been during the initial consultation. He smiled, said hi, and shook my hand.

Sam, my ultimate angel, gave me a reassuring and sympathetic smile. He tried to communicate with his smile that everything was going well and I would be okay. It did comfort me a bit. I got a feeling that I was in safe, responsible, and experienced hands. I had complete faith in the team of experts and that they would do whatever it took to make things turn out well for me.

The nurses were helping in transferring me to the bed. They put a drip in my veins to inject anaesthesia. In a few minutes time, I could feel myself going into a deep sleep and my eyes began to droop. I counted 10, 9,8,7,6... The light in front of my eyes had gone out, and I laid unconscious on the operation table.

It was all dark, just like the way it is when I go to sleep. You would not be able to make out anything in sight. The only difference was the anaesthesia that had worn off and the change of bed.

I had no clue about the duration of the surgery, but I was later told that it had lasted around 6.5 hours. My eyes gave me a direct projection of the ceiling as I opened them after the deep sleep. I was trying to adhere to reality, and I found it difficult for a while to focus.

The staff fussed around me while I was lying motionless on the bed. It was certain that they were all done, and I was thankful for the fact that there had been no complications.

The first thing that came as a sledgehammer was the fact that my whole body was aching. I felt disabled and I felt uncomfortable. I was having a hard time to focus on literally anything. I had felt lightheaded when I first opened my eyes but it was followed by nausea. I could feel numbness throughout my body, and yet I could feel the pain.

If I had to describe what I felt, it was like being a victim of a traffic collision.

With my sight still blurry, I tried to adjust to the brightness in the room. I knew that I would never be the same as before, from the inside and from the outside. My insides had been rearranged and reconstructed.

I would need lots of time to adjust to it. The doctors were delighted to see me awake. The surgery had gone without complications, and the boat I was on had sailed smoothly, at least, up till now. We just had to wait for my healing process to begin.

The entire procedure was done using the key-hole surgery approach, which means that I was plumbed only from the inside and there were no huge scars and cuts on the outside that required too much healing, I only had 6 tiny holes on my tummy area.

I was taken back to the ward and noticed a change. I had an odd feeling, I cannot really describe it, and it was entirely alien. In the semi-conscious state, I was shifted onto my bed, it felt gratifying but even though I was in immense pain, strangely I felt at ease.

I had been stuck in an anaesthesia-induced sleep, and I was cherishing the fact that I still had a bed to lay upon.

I dozed off again. When I woke up, I had a clear head, but the strange feeling remained. Even so, I had greater control of myself. My heart rejoiced about the step I had taken; I had reached another milestone. I was delighted with myself with the first hurdle surpassed.

What had been only words now had been accomplished. It was about time that we all would be able to see visible differences. I really couldn't wait. I wanted to go into a deep sleep, only to wake up when I had become slim and trim. I couldn't think about the hard work and healing to go by.

I was kept under strict observation for the next 72 hours. With the passing days, I felt more in control. I knew that it would take a long time before my body began to comply with the changes done and I began to feel comfortable. I was tired, but felt rejuvenated. A brief check was performed to see if everything was well. On confirmation, I was discharged.

I dressed and met my husband; he was clearly glad to see me trying to keep my mood positive. I was happier to leave the needles and the hospital behind. The hospital was indeed a great one, but I just needed to get home.

It was the start of a new era for me! My girls squealed as I arrived home. I was grateful to God for letting me get here and see them again.

They asked me again and again where had I been and what had happened to me. I continuously told them that I was fine, and it was true. I actually hadn't felt better.

I had to live on liquids and gooey food for the next fourteen days. It was tormenting for me, given the fact that I am someone who loves food. I was far away from enjoying the luxury of 'eating my lovely tasty food.' I was strictly prescribed to eat liquid food; there aren't many options when you come to it.

The options didn't do much justice to my taste buds. The first bite of various foods would leave me feeling disgusted and irritated to the extent that I would want to throw up. I still had to keep up with it, just for the sake of putting something in my stomach.

I was literally longing to eat like a normal person; I never knew that eating like a regular person would become a privilege. One thing was certain, I was only craving and not actually hungry; it was brain hunger. It was just an urge. I had undergone a surgical procedure just a few days back and I couldn't risk my life by eating anything heavy. It could cause damage beyond repair and may also be fatal.

The realisation was strong enough to suppress my cravings for roast chicken for dinner. I had begun to appreciate the times when I could eat whatever I had liked with zero restrictions, zero fears, and zero regrets.

After the first fourteen days, I began to eat marginally more solidified food. It actually came as a relief, and I began to feel more normal. However, I knew one thing, I could never enjoy those rich meals ever again. No doubt, I could eat a relatively normal meal. But everything comes with a sacrifice, and so did my weight reduction. I knew that it was just the beginning of it.

Caution was the key! My meals had to be planned with immense caution. I had to be careful with the fats I consumed. My body was now tailored to not consume enough fats as it had in the past and I had to adjust my eating habits according to it. Only 30% of the fats I consumed before, could be consumed now, the rest would just pass through me, undigested.

How did I know this? Well, I tried it a few times and was left with the worst of stomach aches and toilet issues. This was certainly not to be underestimated. I once had cheese on toast, just 1 slice, and almost didn't make it home from a short shop visit. The pain and urgency 'to go' were intense, and once I had gone to the lavatory, the results were just as bad. The smell and consistency were just horrendous. Things are still the same even now if I go off the rails with my fat intake. My body will only absorb 30% of fat. Anything beyond that just comes away, fast, sometimes with very little time notice given!

I began to see results, and with the amazing results, my regrets of pain and toilet fears began to diminish. The restlessness was turning into excitement. I began to shrink daily as weeks passed. I was like a giant balloon that allowed only a slight amount of air to leave through a slit, and that magical air trimmed me over time. I was deflating!

I maintained a weight loss diary. It began in April 2006 when I lost nearly a stone a month. A stone approximately equals to 14 pounds; and I lost one, and so forth, on a daily, weekly, and monthly basis.

The additional cost we hadn't budgeted for was the fact that I had to keep changing my wardrobe as the old clothes would not fit the new me. It was indeed very costly to buy new things every month, even down to my underwear and shoes! Costly, yet I enjoyed it so much.

I did try and buy lots of low-cost clothing as they wouldn't stay in my wardrobe for long as I continued to shrink. Lots of visits to charity shops for bargains became a regular event. I also dropped a shoe size as well as my waistline. My shrinking feet would make me laugh at different occasions; they looked like a different person's feet when I looked down.

My bra size shrunk too, to no surprise! My hips had grown to approx. 68 inch; they also began to reduce drastically. I could be called "the incredible shrinking woman," and I loved it.

I looked different and thinner every week and I felt awesome! While the weight and size dropped, my self-esteem and confidence grew. I was grateful for it and I was grateful for the fact that I had started to wear less of the boring old clothes.

My weight before had forced me to dress like someone much older than my age and I hadn't liked it at all. Now I was upping my wardrobe game. I could experiment and wear various types of clothing rather than baggy oversized outfits.

When I'd look at what I was becoming in the mirror, at this early stage, I loved it even more. I always had a bright smile on my face. I had a sense of achievement and a constant confidence surge.

I knew that choosing the DS surgery had been the right choice for me. My husband felt like he was with a new woman, and the idea of this new woman was beginning to scare him I think. I had no clue about it. I had completely alienated myself from the emotional effects this could have on my nearest and dearest.

Presumably, he should have felt as excited as I was, and at first, he was. What should have strengthened our bond actually started to crack it.

I remember passing by a shop window once and not recognizing the lady I would see. For a while, I was flabbergasted, but, my shock soon turned into a smile.

Even after so many years, I can remember the change as if it all just happened yesterday. The memory of the bloated woman is still so new that sometimes it becomes hard to believe that so many years have passed.

Just 12 months following surgery, and 13 stone lighter, I met a few of my old friends; they couldn't believe that it was me. A friend said that I looked a decade younger. I looked like a different person, though I was still the same person, but yes, my body had changed so dramatically in just a year.

My co-workers were also shocked due to the drastic change. People also started treating me differently; I was no longer the fat lady, sometimes perceived aggressive, whom everyone would be wary of. I was somehow softer in appearance or just softer on the eyes.

I was sometimes made to feel invisible before, by some people. But now, I had my presence felt. People tended to listen to me more, especially at work.

Anyone that knew of my surgery had their own thoughts about it. Some disregarded my decision and told me off for cheating on diets and exercise and taking the 'easy' option. Others, though, praised me for the commendable decision I took and the huge steps taken over the previous year. Even now, I get mixed opinions; some see it as cheating while others commend me.

My family was always loving and supportive; they treated me in the same way as they had before. They were, at times, worried about my bowel issues and the urgency to use the toilet and due to the pain it would cause me. But they were still highly supportive of me and excited for me.

I would suffer from various sickness episodes, every now and then. It was something that I had literally signed up for. Sometimes, the sickness would strike just because it had to while on other occasions, it would come as a result of high-fat food consumption.

My family dealt with my daily dose of drama while I chose what to eat and what not to. I had to be cautious while dining. The fats would not be absorbed easily while the sugars and carbs would. I also realized that if I only ate carbs I could put back the weight too, which was a point of concern.

So, I had to be extra careful with the food I chose. Feeding on sugars and carbohydrates would mean that I could regain the weight much easily, and I couldn't let that happen. I began to have a high-protein diet, consisting of meats and fish along with veg-salads.

I had never experienced such a diet before! I could eat bread, but that too in modest quantity, as it could upset my tummy, and I also became lactose intolerant. I was forced to follow the diet. Failing to comply could result in me gaining all the weight that I had shed or else, spending hours in the toilet with immense pain and inconvenience – that was the worst side effect.

I would be forced to spend hours in the toilet even, at work, and this would make me reflect upon the fact that wouldn't everyone wonder where have I gone?

It made me more cautious about my eating habits. I couldn't let the horrendous results take over my health and my life.

With trials, errors and sufferings; I got the hang of my body's needs and began to adjust likewise. However, my temptations would win sometimes, and I'd treat myself with junk food, and my stomach would make me pay for it. Massive pain and loose oily stools would be uncontrollable.

Determination, dedication, and time; these three things taught me how to go about this new diet and maintain my eating habits.

The element of mal-absorption had to be taken into account, as well. I had yet to figure out ways to keep the vitamin and nutrients level intact; I was taking supplements to ensure to keep my levels normal or else, I could suffer from malnutrition. This was one of the main risks of the DS surgery that I'd signed up for.

Everything has a price and what I traded for food was something tremendously important. If you think I've begun to regret it, no, not at all.

It gave me so much that I'm highly grateful for. I became an entirely different woman physically. I looked more desirable! Also, healthier. I would go swimming with my girls and it definitely made me more flexible and energetic.

There was another thing which didn't fit in the frame well, my loose skin. The fat reduced, dramatically, but my skin didn't shrink; at least not at the same rate.

In some areas, it shrunk steadily, while it showed stubbornness in other areas. It didn't shrink at all, skin just hung.

My skin became increasingly saggy, it made me look ugly and old, and I didn't like it. It was worse than the fat had made me feel.

This weight reduction regime wasn't working like I thought it would. I had presumed that my weight would reduce and the skin would shrink, but the reality was far from it. Actually, if I'm honest I never really thought about the excess skin I'd be left with.

Now, this was another problem that was yet to be dealt with. I was still adjusting my eating habits and accepting a new way of living. This was something that could make my bubble of joy to burst, and this was the last thing that I had wanted to happen.

In true terms, I was becoming a deflated balloon, with a lot of loose skin. I had to get rid of all that **extra** skin and what did it call for? More surgery, more cost? Sadly YES!

~End of chapter 2~

## Chapter 3: Saggy skin!! What's next?

As the years passed, the weight loss surgery caused me many more medical issues, which required a lot of understanding and support, plus more surgery and medication – the pain was certainly not over yet, in fact just starting.

Twelve months had passed, and things were certainly not the same as before. They were drastically different from the time when I had first undergone the surgical procedures. I had lost approx. 13 stones of weight at approx. at 170lbs, but the blessing came with a curse as well, i.e., the awful saggy skin.

It became a major issue for me. Every time I'd look in the mirror to cherish my transformation, I'd be forced to notice something that I hated. My skin didn't shrink with the pace of my weight loss, and it made me look utterly awful.

I began to despair regarding my decision. Every time I'd look at myself in the mirror, a part of my heart would ache. This wasn't something that I was looking forward to initially. I just didn't see that coming. I knew it wasn't going to be easy, but I didn't know that it was going to be like this! I'd look like an old lady, naked. The feeling was worse than it had been before when I was fat.

The thrill of losing weight had begun to diminish. The moment I began to love my body, the sagging skin appeared to destroy it all. My body was at its worst. Saggy breasts, saggy thighs, saggy arms, and saggy everything! The only pleasant parts in my entire body were my face and my neck, which had retained their tightness, thank goodness.

I used to look like I was in my 50s before when I was fat, but now I looked like a 90-year-old, while only being in my early 30s. I looked like a recently popped balloon, and I was obviously not okay with it.

Was I wanting too much?

People had been complimenting me for my weight loss, which was great as most of my saggy skin was hidden. I wore clothes which would cover my entire body, just to make sure that none of my loose skin showed. As a result, people didn't notice if something was wrong. On other occasions, if someone would catch a glimpse of my arms or any other body part, it would make me feel just awful.

Getting undressed and then dressed was a task that in and of itself made me feel pathetic about my body! I really couldn't muster the courage to look down on my hanging flabby legs and stomach. It was daunting. You just cannot separate yourself from your body, and I began to hate it again, even more than before.

I had been dealing with this situation for over a year now! I remember the shattering task of folding my small saggy boobs into my bra to make them look in some kind of acceptable shape. My cleavage would look rather laughable because it wasn't something that could be shown off anymore, it was all wrinkled and empty. I started wearing clothes which covered me up to my shoulders. My body was covered with stretch marks, wrinkles, and saggy skin. Their accumulation was a big turn off for me, and I'm sure for my husband.

I had to keep my entire body covered. I could only see two things in my body, unattractiveness, and ugliness. I had become a disaster, and this would keep me worried all the time. It deteriorated all aspects of my life; my husband and I just stopped talking and doing things together. I felt so low.

I developed a habit of taking my clothes into the bathroom in order to change or on other occasions I'd wake up early to take a bath or shower, so I wouldn't be seen. I was not ready to accept my body as it is. My body looked far better and beautiful when I had tons of fat on it. How had I been so ignorant of the skin I'd be left with?

I had been tremendously happy with my initial weight loss, and I was so excited to embrace my new body. I did this all for what I thought were the right reasons. But now I knew that I had wanted to just to look and feel 'normal'.

I took refuge in the internet once again. I began to do some research. Just like before. It pointed me in the direction of reconstruction surgery; it was amazing that no one had spoken to me about this stage, not the dietician at the hospital or my surgeon, Sam, no one.

To be content with myself and stay happy in the future, I had to go through more surgical procedures, and I knew that it would be pricey.

I literally needed a tummy tuck to rid myself of the 20 inches of loose skin on my stomach; my legs and arms also needed work along with my breasts.

I couldn't afford to get the procedures done in the United Kingdom. I began to search for alternates outside of the UK. The prices abroad were much lower. I came across a competent and well-established surgeon in Prague who could do this for me. I reached out for reviews from his patients. I couldn't take risks, not with finance and not with my life, so I did my homework!

I got the "before and after" pictures from the patients and asked the questions that mattered. The research and reviews provided me with a confirmation that I should go ahead with this surgeon.

The best part about the procedure with him was that it would cost less than 3<sup>rd</sup> of what I would pay in the United Kingdom. It seemed like a perfect package; it came with a cheaper price quotation and an ideal body goal along with positive recommendations from other patients.

I reached out to the surgeon in Prague, and we discussed the procedures over the phone. I explicitly told him that I needed to get everything tucked in desperately. From belly to breasts, from legs to arms; literally everything, I also sent him lots of pictures of my body.

I was longing to see my skin become like any normal person's. I wanted to stay happy without hiding so much of my skin under big clothes again. The surgeon told me that all of this could not be done in one visit, but in a number of visits.

All this hanging skin had to be cut away in stages. This would give my body the best chance to heal and to avoid too much pain and stress.

As per his advice, I opted for a breast lift and a tummy tuck as my first preference. I couldn't opt for my arms because I'd need them fit and healthy to provide lifting support to me post this first surgery.

I was lucky that I had a well-paying job. It allowed me to have some savings of my own. I could make use of them during this next step of my journey.

The tough part was talking about this with my friends and family. They had been very supportive the entire time, and they loved me with or without the ton of loose skin.

Their main concern was seeing me in immense pain once again, let alone the financial burden it would impose on hubby and me.

As for me, the journey that I had set foot on wasn't complete and couldn't be completed without the reconstruction surgery.

The feelings I had at this point were strange and not as exciting as before. I was nervous and worried. I was going to a different country, so it would be a completely new experience.

Although scared, I was determined. I believed that everything would turn out well, and this was just another stage in this journey.

On the day when I boarded my flight, I had constant thoughts of cancelling the trip. These thoughts remained with me until I reached a point of no return, i.e., until I had already boarded and I sat alone on the plane.

The journey gave me chills. A dark and unfamiliar car was waiting for me at the airport in Prague. As I got in, I saw a man inside who greeted me. He drove me to my destination. During the car journey, I tried nervously to make conversation with him. But he barely uttered a word and just kept nodding.

The car drove me out of the busy streets of this beautiful city into a quieter yet more peaceful part of the suburbs. I clutched my handbag tightly and was continuously texting my husband. The car then pulled in front of a remote white building. I stepped out of the car, and so did the driver. He escorted me into the building where my preliminary medical checks were performed and then back in that awful car again to the main clinic.

There was a huge linguistic barrier. I could see only two nurses and no patients in sight. The walls were pristine and white. The clinic was silent like that of morgue behind closed doors, but it smelled clean and was spotless.

It was more clean and hygienic than any of the hospitals in the UK I'd visited... He led me into a room where I was asked to sit.

After a short wait, I saw the surgeon. He discussed the procedures with me and then the staff was instructed to prepare me for my surgery the very next day. His English was very good, was and that made me relaxed.

The next day the surgeon came in, followed by his team. He asked me if I had slept well and was comfortable. I told him the truth that I felt at ease.

They continued to relax. I was awed by the overall layout and the professional approach that the clinic followed. Everything was set exactly in place.

I felt that I was in good hands and extremely safe. The surgeon began to draw lines on the parts he was going to cut. I felt like a life-sized drawing board.

He took me to the room where the surgery was to be performed. There were two nurses who smiled and nodded as I went inside. They prepared me for the procedure.

I was injected with anaesthesia and fell into a deep sleep, with obvious hope and prayers that everything would turn out just perfect. Although I didn't quite know what to expect this time.

When I woke up, I was in toe-curling pain! I thought that something had gone wrong. What had I done to myself?

The nurses helped me with the pain. The pain I had to endure when I got the DS surgical procedures back in the United Kingdom was peanuts in contrast to what I was feeling at that time. This was literally like I'd been cut in half. I couldn't get up. I couldn't move. I felt like I had been sliced up. I had this feeling of tightness and confinement all over my body. As I tried to move my arms, I couldn't move them higher than above my waist, my body was so tight.

I just lay on my bed, trying to relax and kill time, thinking and hoping that all of this would end soon and I'd have a very speedy recovery. I could already feel that my breasts were in good shape now. I felt that I had done the right thing. They weren't saggy at all and were strapped up tightly. They were swollen and very sore but felt at least as if they were in the right place.

I had also asked for a small sized implant in addition to the lifting and augmentation. I felt they were okay and the right size albeit swollen.

My tummy was so sore though. My body was kept high on morphine, and I kept dozing off from time to time. Despite being pumped full of drugs, I could still feel traces of pain.

However, the staff were extremely helpful, and they took really good care of me.

I stayed for a few days at the clinic, and the staff kept a thorough check on me. They would put me through a routine check-up daily and kept me topped up with pain killers.

Now that I was through these surgical procedures. I was eager to look at myself in the mirror. I would leave it a few weeks though until the healing had progressed.

I knew that I had a long way to go. There was much still to be done; my arms and my legs still needed work. I reminded myself that this could not be done before I had healed well. I felt the finish line was in sight, again.

After a few days in the hospital, I was allowed to board a flight back home. Something awful happened during the flight. My breasts began to swell and throb. It frightened me to death. The first thought that came into my mind was that they had done a bad job which was so frightening, I thought my breasts would explode any time.

I didn't want to imagine how horrendous it would be if my thoughts turned into reality.

To my relief, the bloating subsided. I thought this was just normal and I ignored it; it was my optimism guiding me, as ever. I took the journey back home, on my own. My husband was home and had looked after my girls during the process. They were all there when I got back, I was so relieved to be back home albeit, in pain, I felt secure and safe.

Now my diet included a handful of painkillers as well since the pain had yet to subside. I stayed off work for nearly six weeks. There was no way that I could manage going to work during this time.

I took this time as an opportunity to rest; I literally needed it. My body felt like it had been chewed up. The turmoil I was feeling was something that I was experiencing for the first time.

This time, it was much tougher. The movement became harder; I was forced to walk slowly and could hardly lean and bend. That being said, you know how kids are; my little girls would walk and run so fast. My husband told them that mummy wasn't well and they needed to help in taking care of mummy.

I kept on going; I tried my best to get well, as soon as possible. As I recovered, I began to ponder over the next step.

I was in love with the job that had been done on my breasts and my tummy, and I just wanted to make the rest of my body look this good too.

Though I hadn't completely recovered, I was looking forward to my upcoming surgeries. With six weeks gone, I felt much better. With minimal pain, my scars also were healing well. I was beginning to look forward to booking my next surgery session.

The tight feeling in my stomach had reduced, and I was able to put the girls to bed just like I did before.

Everything was returning to its place, my optimism too. Then, during one afternoon at home, my left breast began to ache. It started just like the same pain that I had experienced on my way back from Prague. But then it very quickly became much worse.

My left breast continued to swell uncontrollably. It just wouldn't stop. It grew and swelled literally growing to under my chin. It swelled so big, like a football. I was terrified! I hadn't seen any such thing happen to anyone before, nor had I ever heard about it being a side effect. I didn't know what to do, panic took over.

My heart skipped beats; I thought I was going to die. Would my longing for a perfect body finally take my life, after all I'd been through so far?

We immediately called for an ambulance, and I was rushed to the nearest hospital. I cried during the entire journey. The pain was immense, and it felt like that breast would explode at any time. My husband had to stay back home with my girls again. I felt alone and terrible with the thought of dying in this state of emergency, without my loved ones – all alone.

After lots of tests, a big blood clot was discovered in my left breast, and it had to be treated quickly. The surgeon said that they might even take out the implant. This got me very worried.

I wondered if they will only take the implant out of one of my breasts or both. This experience was utterly awful. They took me to the emergency operating room; I was constantly asking myself what would happen.

How had this happened? Why did I risk my life just for a better body!

The surgery continued for two hours. I opened my eyes from the induced sleep.

The surgeon gave me the good news. He said that he had managed to save the breast and had cleaned out the cavity and removed the blood clot. I now had to recover emotionally and physically. This situation had been traumatic. I spent weeks in the hospital trying to recuperate from that experience.

Something that scared more was the fact that if the clot had reached to my lungs, I was told, I could have been inches from death.

I contacted my doctor in Prague and updated him about my situation. He was concerned about my health, and I assured him that I was doing perfectly fine and was recovering well.

He offered to pay for a return flight so that I could visit him and he could make sure that all is well.

I turned him down. I told him that I was all good. The disaster had been cared for, and thus there was no point in visiting him.

As everything began to go back to its normal shape, my desire for the rest of the reconstructive work came back once again. I was actually looking forward to my arm and thigh surgery, as that would be the end.

Six months went by. I had recovered in the entirety, so I then returned to Prague. It was just the same – all of it like last time, i.e., the same driver, the same professionalism, the same car, and the same building.

My doctor was happy to see me, specifically after the drama that had happened to me before.

I was more content this time. I knew that my choice was correct. I was all set for the second procedure.

But I was wrong. I thought that the pain I felt during the tummy tuck was the worst that could ever happen. However, after the second procedure, I saw new levels of pain.

The worst part was that my arms and thighs had to be used in making most movements, and they couldn't be put totally at rest like the other parts of my body could.

The pain was immense! I spent a few days in the hospital and then returned back home, alone, once again. The flab had finally gone. I kept on thinking about the possibility of never getting rid of them and this haunted me.

That being said, I was relieved that I didn't have to get any nipping and tucking done on my face and neck since they hadn't become too saggy, I always looked great from the neck upwards! Was it really over, finally? It would have been terribly painful if the same procedure was done on my face, and honestly, I feel blessed regarding that.

When I look back and reflect upon what had happened, I know one thing: I was horror-struck when my breasts began to swell, which was separate from any procedure I'd had done...

I don't regret any of the reconstruction performed. It made a huge difference in my life and my overall wellbeing. And honestly, I needed it. It gave me a sense of starting a whole new life. It gave me new beginnings. What I have learned is that the two procedures go hand in hand. You cannot go for just the weight loss surgery alone, without following it with reconstructive work.

Ask yourself could you live with pounds of saggy skin and be pleased with your weight loss surgery? Obviously not! I have to admit, I had set foot on this journey half-prepared. I hadn't known the full consequences; neither did I know anything about the REAL costs, either physically, financially or emotionally.

Above all, no one had told me about the pain that I would have to endure. It came as something utterly unexpected. I had known that the procedures would be painful, but not in a way that I'd feel like I'd die due to it!

I had dealt with depression, diet changes, and a complete lifestyle shift. But it was all worth it! When I look at myself in the mirror today, I am proud of the person I see. I am proud of my choice, and I know that I did the right thing.

However, I am also happy that it's over. I have scars on my body, but they aren't aberrations. They tell my story. I can see them on my naked body now, but they're fading.

I would never want to go through all of it again, ever in my life! I have maintained a kind of discipline in my life, and I don't plan to gain any kind of weight in any way. But I don't regret doing what I did.

The best advice that I have for anyone is, "Don't get fat in the first instance!" That's because you will have to pay for it in the long run. Prevention is always better than a cure.

As soon as the healing procedure sped up, I felt more confident in mingling with people, and in myself. No one could see my saggy skin anymore. It was all gone, and I felt great. However, while I began to enjoy a positive position in my other relationships, my marital life had suffered. It had been tarnished beyond repair, not through any fault on either part.

Both of us really couldn't see the problems and the issues we have had before. Maybe we were too blind and always had accepted things as they were.

We separated on good terms. He is an amazing friend even to date and has been the best dad for my girls. We both needed and wanted more from our relationship. We wanted different things, just not from each other.

If I try to describe it, I just can't! We were together, living happily, like friends. But we weren't meant to be together as man and wife. There was some kind of silence between us. I am very grateful for his support. I couldn't have done this without him. He was always my rock giving me support and comfort along this journey…

We tried to mend the issues in our relationship, but it didn't work. We were both suffering emotionally. We couldn't live like a couple anymore. We decided to part ways. However, we shall always be good friends, as we have 2 beautiful girls.

We are still very close, and he always goes that extra mile for my daughters. He never disappoints as a father. You may think that my pursuit of a new body made me lose my closest relationship, but this is not the case.

We just weren't meant to be.

I am now living a happier life with my new man. We have been together for over 14 years now, and I hope that we never get to meet the fat Jo again!

~End of chapter 3~

# Chapter 4: The New Me…FOURTEEN Years plus

Over fourteen years down the road, I am now in a place where I feel content with the way I look and feel. When I had started my journey to a new me, I knew it would require significant life changes from my side. But I had also understood that I must make it happen because I also wanted to be healthier and fitter for my young family.

When you have kids, your routine changes, gone is the personal or 'me' time that you used to have. Consequently, you exercise less and focus on your diet even lesser. It is all about getting things done in time, for example, making sure the kids reach school on time or dinner's ready, washing is done, the house is clean, etc. The result can often result in complacency, which can cause the weight to keep piling on, plus juggling huge work and home commitments is tough too.

One of the physical changes that I am most happy about is that I am healthier and able to spend more time with my kids. I do things that I couldn't have done before. Physical exertion didn't just exhaust my body before, it also left me mentally exhausted. But the new me can be a part of my kids' life to a more significant extent, and I enjoy what they enjoy doing.

I have also made emotional strides. My self-confidence has increased, and I am proud of the way I look and feel. A mental belief that after everything I have been through, I managed to come out on top and I am satisfied with who I am now.

I am a happier and more vibrant person. I am amazed at how the way I look has changed the way I look at the world. I feel good both inside and outside. Discovering that I am open to new experiences is completely opposite to the way I used to feel.

When I think about the journey that brought me to where I am now, I realize how arduous it was. I put my body through a lot of stress, and my mind wasn't under any less strain. I had a long and tough time – both physically and mentally – to get here.

So, would I change anything about the way things happened before? Would I spare myself the pain and the anguish that I went through? Absolutely, if I had a magic wand! Although, I wouldn't have learned the same valuable lessons that I did if the change had come easy.

I also wouldn't value life the way I do right now. Each pound that I lost was the result of a huge struggle, albeit a different struggle to the normal way of losing weight. Every scar on my body due to the surgeries I went through, isn't just a mark. It is the evidence of my battles, and procedures that I fought and ultimately won.

I was fighting for a better life. To live longer and to be able to spend more time with my daughters. I was fighting for a new me who would be satisfied with the way she looked and felt. Each time I went under the knife, my tenacity only strengthened. I was going to make it, and I was going to come out of this stronger than before. And that is exactly what I did. I'm just glad I'm at the other side looking in.

However, my success hasn't come without a cost. It isn't just what I went through in the past that has been difficult. My life still isn't easy because of the constant pain that challenges my body. I have to be consistent when it comes to the many ongoing daily medications that I must take. The weight loss surgery left behind a barrage of both outside and inside health issues.

My daily regime consists of taking an array of tablets daily. These include various vitamins and minerals that keep my body strong and functional. I take folic acid, iron, and calcium supplements every day.

Besides that, I was also diagnosed with a bone disorder, Osteoporosis, a few years after my weight loss surgery. That's another reason that I have to maintain a daily intake of calcium. Calcium is good for bone and teeth strength.

Osteoporosis is a condition where bones can begin to lose their density. Consequently, they are easier to break and fracture. People with osteoporosis need to be very careful when they move. Any bumps or falls can result in fractures or bone breakage.

There's a limit to how much I can exercise and the kinds of exercises that I can do as well. Anything that would strain my spine is a big No, No.

I have also noticed changes in the way I move, both consciously and subconsciously. For instance, now when I bend, my body doesn't bend in the same way that it used to before I was diagnosed with Osteoporosis.

The movement that was hard for me because of my weight before the surgery has become difficult for me due to this bone disorder.

Since my body doesn't respond the way it should, given that I weigh much less now, I have to be careful when doing household chores. For instance, I divide my ironing into several batches. That way, I don't put undue strain on my back, which can be dangerous. It took some getting used to, but I have learned how to manage myself now and continue with a busy life.

Besides my difficulties with Osteoporosis, I am also dealing with another post-operative disorder. Recently, I was diagnosed with Fibromyalgia. If you are unfamiliar with this, try to imagine feeling tired and being in pain most of the time. My health issues have become a real concern for me. After being diagnosed with fibromyalgia, life is harder due to fatigue, physical weakness, and pain. I'm not sure if it has to do with weight loss surgery or not, but I do feel weaker and less strong because of it.

Every morning I wake up and then roll over onto one side slowly. Then using my arm to lift me, I sit up in bed. Only then I can attempt to get up. If I try sitting up first from a lying position, I end up hurting and feeling so much pain.

Similarly, even when attempting some light activity, I have to do it slowly. That means doing it one step at a time. I can't lift the mattress up, so most of the time, I will leave the blankets and sheets untucked when making the beds. Squatting down to lift something up could put extra strain on my knees, but it's better for my back.

Even now, I forget and try to stand up suddenly or attempt to get out of bed as soon as I have woken up. But most of the time, I remember to take things a bit slower. The pain reminds me of taking things slowly

I am treating Osteoporosis as a learning experience too. The first and most important lesson that I have learned as a result of this disorder is how to set boundaries. By that I mean, I am now confident enough to differentiate between my own values and that of other people. Before this, distinguishing the two was difficult for me, I only push myself to what I can do and not beyond.

Saying no in order to protect myself didn't come easy to me. I now find the time to focus on myself and take care of myself better.

Therefore, I have learned my lesson and always schedule some "me" time for myself. Just like I schedule important dates and appointments on my calendar, I have started setting emotional and physical boundaries. I can tell you that it has helped me tremendously.

What does it mean to have some me time? It means to dedicate a few hours a week to do what you enjoy doing. Whether it is taking up a hobby or by joining a class, doing what we love keeps both physically and mentally healthy.

Incidentally, what I am most passionate about is spending time with my family. An hour or two spent with my kids and new hubby along with my two dogs can be therapeutic in ways I had never imagined before. So, this has only brought me closer to them.

Besides that, I often indulge in other types of self-care. With my newfound confidence, I can go out and spend some time getting my nails done. I love pampering myself and relaxing with a mini facial or massage.

Another aspect of self-care has been for me to eat healthier. Once I started taking care of what I eat, I also started making healthy food for the rest of my family. I have come to realize that I am worth making an extra effort. If that means going on a short walk every now and then to get some exercise, then so be it. I even do yoga now, which I love. Drinking any type of alcohol has had to reduce significantly too due the effect it has on my body, I have been hospitalised with Pancreatitis 4 times, which means I have to either quit fully or suffer the consequences, this is an ongoing battle I face, and struggle with the temptation.

Of course, I have to also take some precautions because of Osteoporosis when it comes to exercise. I, deliberately, keep the walks short. If I feel like exercising in some other manner, I do that by light stretching. I follow it with some meditation, which I have learned now and enjoy to do it regularly.

I have also come to realise that certain people can be very judgemental. Their negativity can be contagious, which is why I gradually try to reduce time with anyone that could affect me badly. By taking care of myself, I can take care of my family more.

I wouldn't change a thing about the whole process I have been through. It has helped me grow as a person. Before, I was quite depressed. My weight was a huge concern for me, although no-one would ever have guessed it with the way I behaved, it was the obsession with being fat that was also taking me away from more important things.

After I achieved the impossible, hopefully, my slimmer body will serve as a good example to my daughters. Growing up with a slimmer mum who feels younger and more positive is a better experience for them.

# In Summary

This isn't just a book; it is a map of the journey that I call a segment of my life! There are triumphs, such as when I overcame my weight affliction against all the odds and changed everything for the better. But you will also see that I had to deal with huge disappointments. I didn't let the adversities stop me, not at all! I pushed on until I had been through multiple surgeries and consistently ate healthy enough to be where I am today.

My previous husband was one of my strongest supporters throughout this ordeal. I'm so pleased that was an amicable ending. My daughters have strong & tenacious role models to look up to in him, plus my new husband, and I hope they take some positivity from my story too as they live their own lives!

I am a fighter, and that remains true even today. Having defeated obesity successfully, I am now battling two further disorders i.e., Fibromyalgia and Osteoporosis. I know I will prevail in the end, and keep going.

I always do!

# My Photographical Transformation

## Pre-Surgery

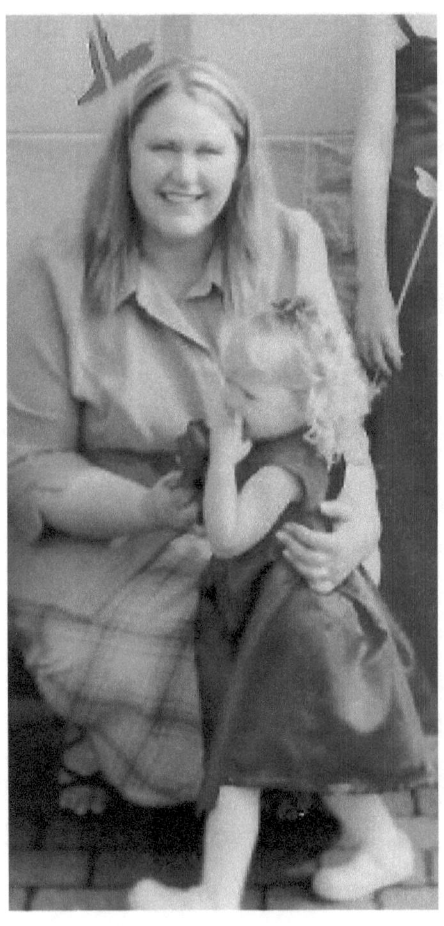

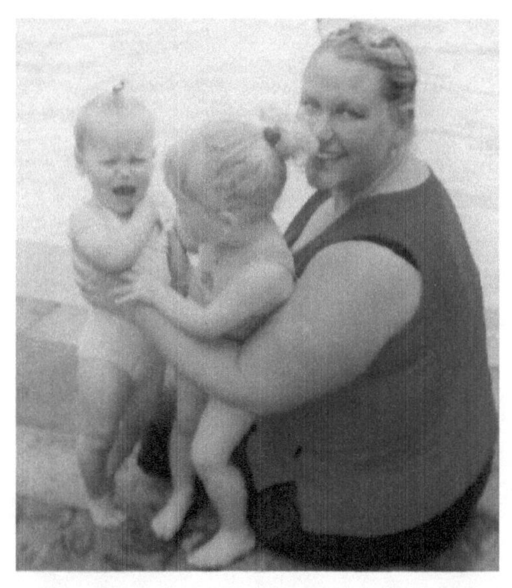

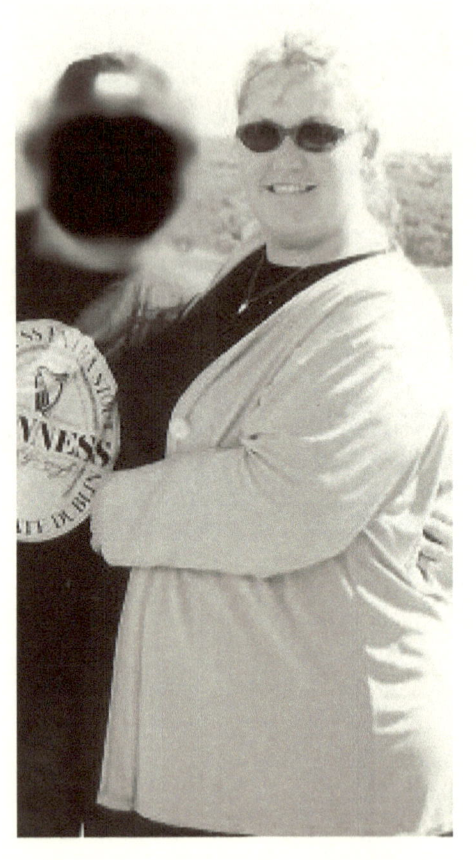

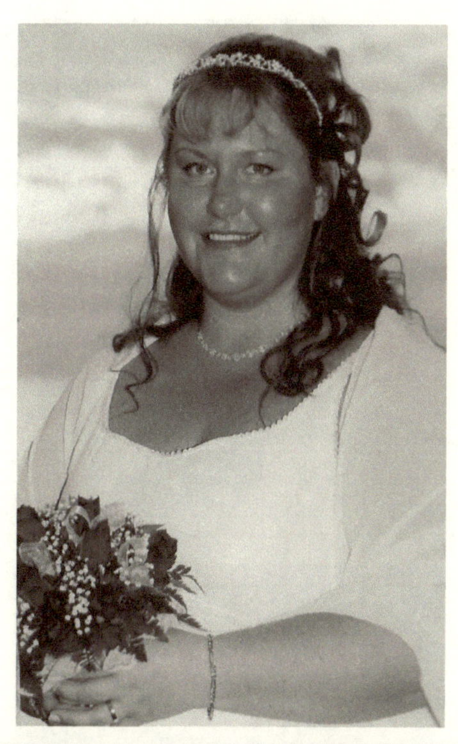

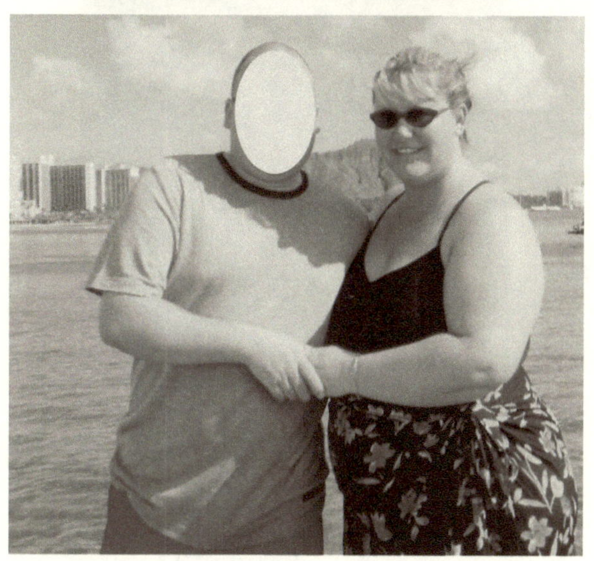

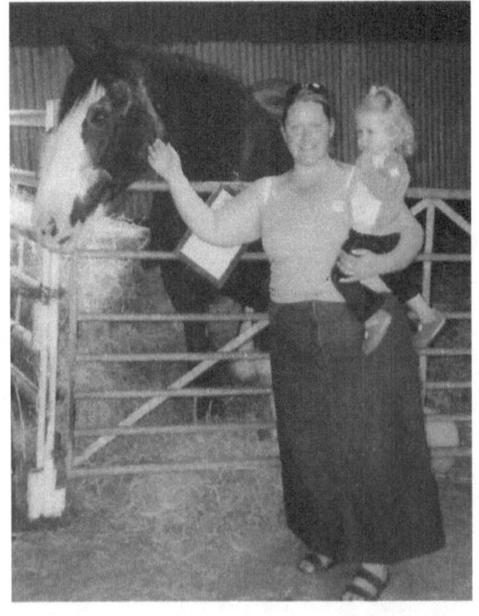

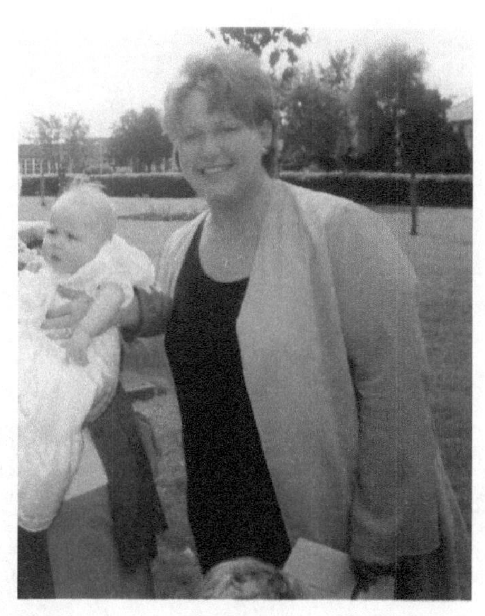

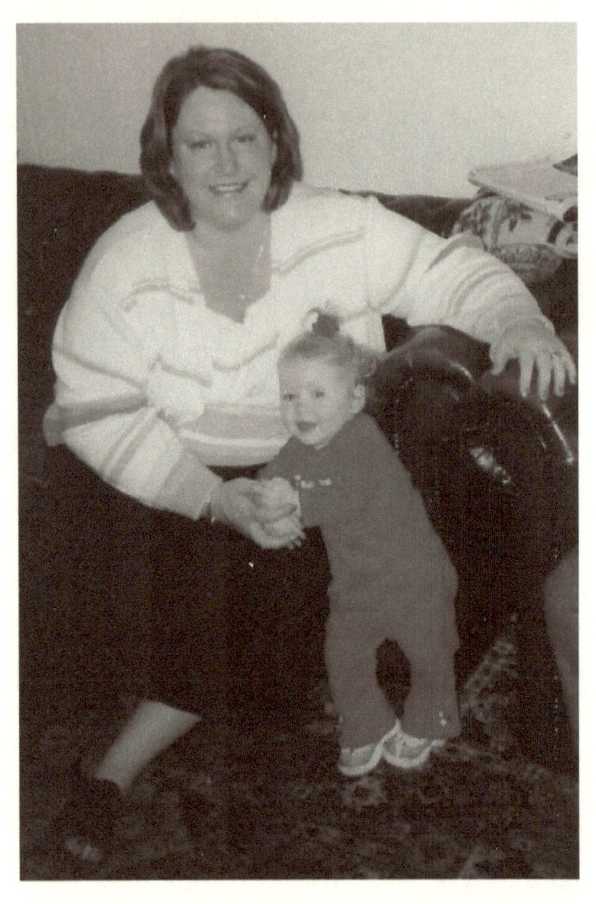

# Post-Surgery

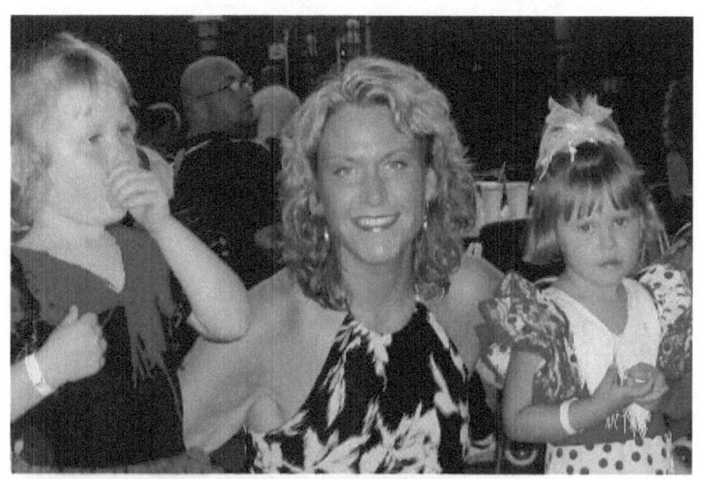

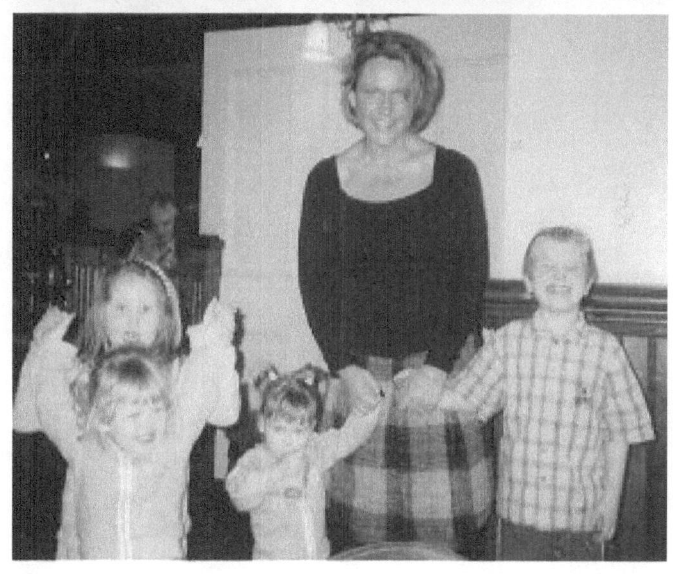

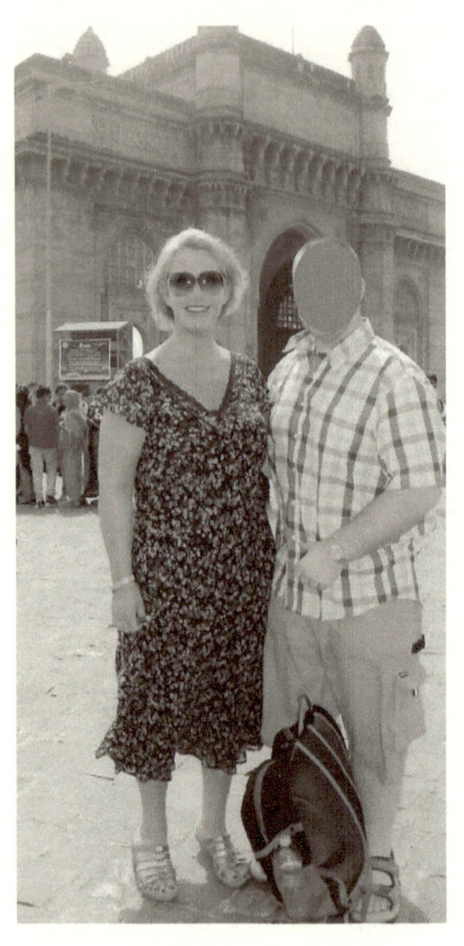

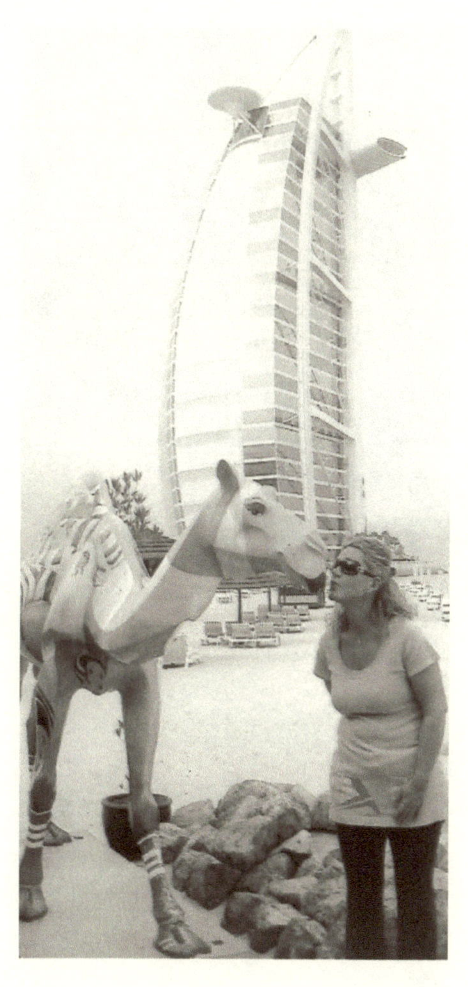

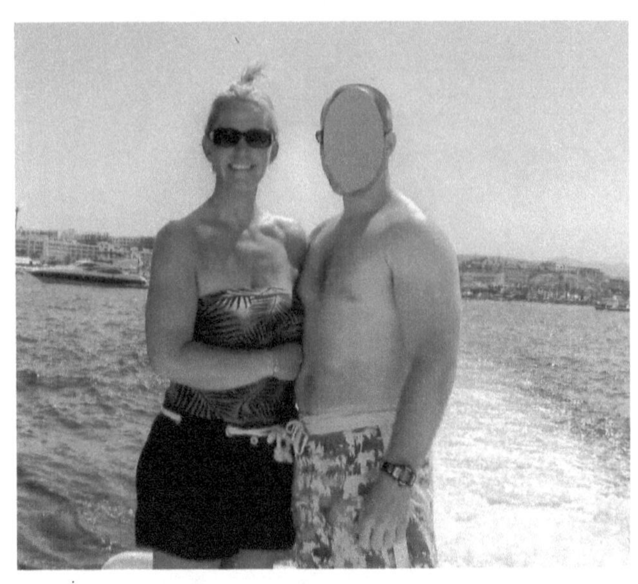

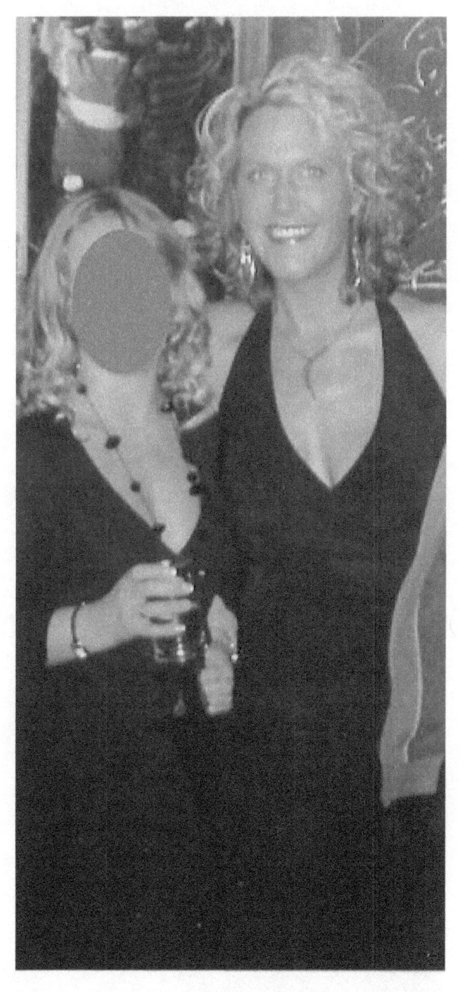

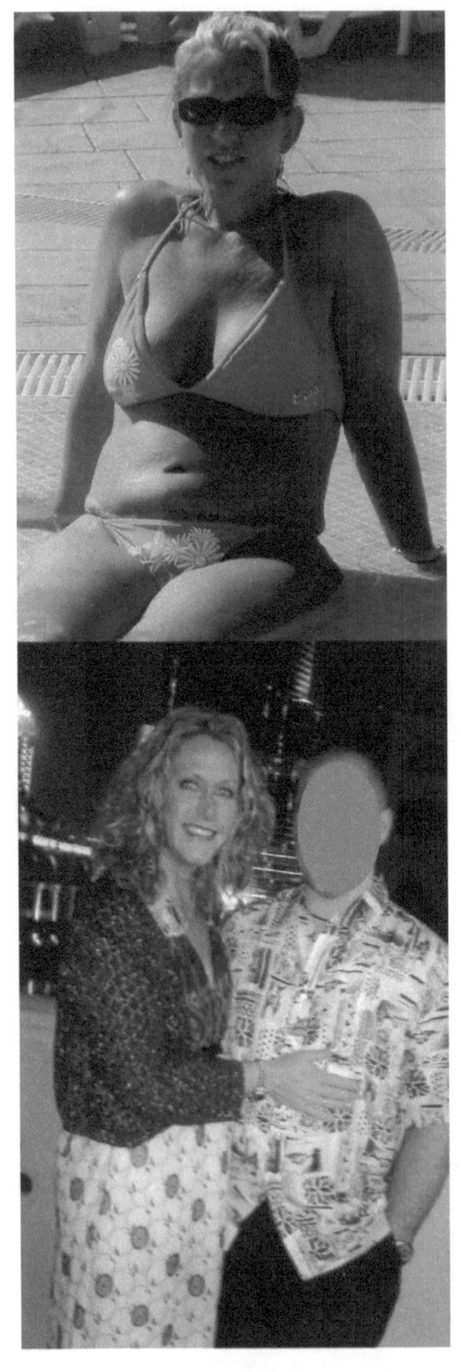

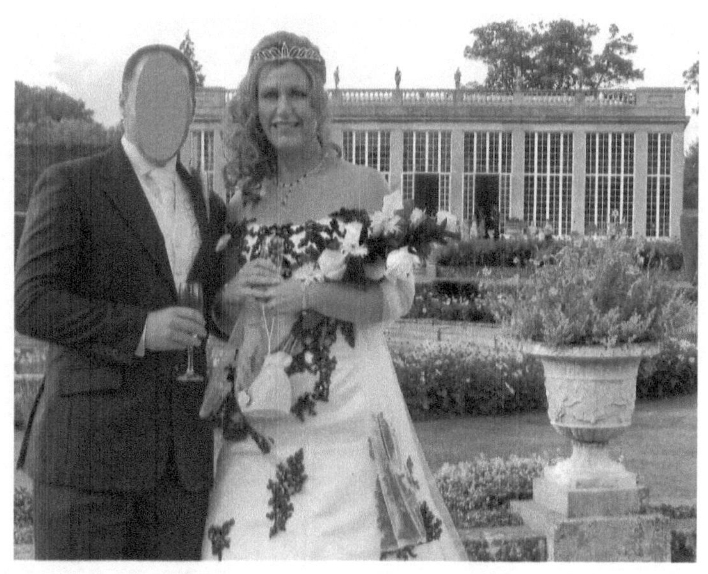